# THE UNIVERSITY
# OF CANCER

# THE UNIVERSITY OF CANCER

### NO ONE APPLIES
### THE CURRICULUM CAN KILL YOU
### THE EDUCATION IS PRICELESS

# JAMES PERRY

Printed in the United States of America.

ISBN Paperback: 978-1-7349196-0-8
ISBN Hardover: 978-1-7349196-1-5
ISBN eBook: 978-1-7349196-2-2

# DEDICATION

This book is dedicated to two of the toughest, most beautiful ladies in my world. Both of them are two-time survivors of cancer. One experienced cancer first in her beloved twenty-three-year-old son and then in her husband of twenty-eight years, both diagnosed within four months and five days of each other. The other experienced cancer with her big brother and her popa, both when she was only nineteen years old. Although these two beautiful ladies never actually had cancer, both had to deal with cancer of their beloved father, husband, son, and brother.

### To my bride, Shanna Lou.

Shanna has spent her life in the most challenging and rewarding career she could have. She is an exceptional wife and mother, part-time pediatric nurse, hematologist, orthopedic specialist, urologist, oncologist, radiologist, taxi driver, Google research expert, chief cook, and bottle washer. She does all this stuff without pay. Her beloved son Julian was diagnosed with cancer when he was twenty-three years old. No one in Shanna's family or my family had ever experienced cancer; this was all new to us.

Shanna has a deep faith and trust in her Lord and would learn what it would be like to lean on Him heavily. Julian was diagnosed on June 5, called his mom, and said, "Mom, I have cancer. Don't worry. I am scheduled for surgery tomorrow morning. Can you get me to the hospital by 5:30 tomorrow morning?" Imagine the emotion that would go through a mother's heart and mind if she were to hear something like that from her son? Shanna was an emotional mess! She had to pull her car over as she was driving down the road to gather herself.

Julian asked her to go to the pharmacy, to get a prescription he needed to take that evening before the surgery. When Shanna was at the pharmacy, she bumped into a friend. Her friend immediately noticed that something was seriously wrong and asked Shanna if everything was all right. Shanna uttered the words for the first time in her life, "My son has cancer!"

She was with him through his surgery and cared for him the way only a mom can. But Julian had a new wife, and Shanna had to learn how to stay out of the way, even when her son had cancer. Julian endured a surgery and four weeks of twenty-five to thirty hours each week of chemotherapy.

Within two weeks of Julian's fourth round of chemotherapy, her husband was diagnosed with cancer. How does someone summon the strength and emotional fortitude to endure and deal with such a life-altering sequence of events?

**To my baby girl, Alexandra Grace.**

When she was born, her mom gave her that middle name, Grace. It is a good thing she did because Alexandra has a gracefulness about her that is evident the moment you come into contact with her. Alexandra not only endured seeing her brother and her father deal with cancer surgeries and miserable treatments, she somehow loved on and encouraged her new sister-in-law Woo Jin and her mom. She spent a lot of time comforting and sharing with Shanna during a tough time and kept her mom from having a nervous breakdown. In a lot of ways, Alexandra displayed a courageous strength and peace that Shanna simply couldn't.

Alexandra spent hours with her brother and her father during doctor trips and chemo treatments. She comforted and was a dear friend, sister, and daughter, not only to Shanna and Woo Jin, but also to Julian and me. She somehow selflessly took on the responsibility of holding our family together, and she did it voluntarily, gracefully, and lovingly. All the while, her brother and Popa had cancer.

These ladies are not only beautiful and inspiring, they are tough chicks! For a better and more thorough understanding of the character and discipline of these two ladies, I invite you to read the thirty-first chapter of the book of Proverbs, verses 10–31 (NIV). There you will find a perfect description of these two beautiful ladies.

# THE WIFE OF NOBLE CHARACTER

A wife of noble character who can find?
　　She is worth far more than rubies.
Her husband has full confidence in her
　　and lacks nothing of value.
She brings him good, not harm,
　　all the days of her life.
She selects wool and flax
　　and works with eager hands.
She is like the merchant ships,
　　bringing her food from afar.
She gets up while it is still night;
　　she provides food for her family
　　and portions for her female servants.
She considers a field and buys it;
　　out of her earnings she plants a vineyard.

She sets about her work vigorously;
    her arms are strong for her tasks.
She sees that her trading is profitable,
    and her lamp does not go out at night.
In her hand she holds the distaff
    and grasps the spindle with her fingers.
She opens her arms to the poor
    and extends her hands to the needy.
When it snows, she has no fear for her household;
    for all of them are clothed in scarlet.
She makes coverings for her bed;
    she is clothed in fine linen and purple.
Her husband is respected at the city gate,
    where he takes his seat among the elders of the land.
She makes linen garments and sells them,
    and supplies the merchants with sashes.
She is clothed with strength and dignity;
    she can laugh at the days to come.
She speaks with wisdom,
    and faithful instruction is on her tongue.
She watches over the affairs of her household
    and does not eat the bread of idleness.
Her children arise and call her blessed;
    her husband also, and he praises her:
"Many women do noble things,
    but you surpass them all."

Charm is deceptive, and beauty is fleeting;
    but a woman who fears the Lord is to be praised.
Honor her for all that her hands have done,
    and let her works bring her praise at the city gate.

God bless you, Shanna and Alexandra.
You inspire me.

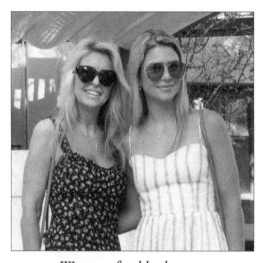

*Women of noble character.*
*Shanna Perry and Alexandra Perry.*

# CONTENTS

**Preface** . . . . . . . . . . . . . . . . . . . . . . . . . . . . . . . . . xv

**Introduction** . . . . . . . . . . . . . . . . . . . . . . . . . . . . . 1

**No One Applies** . . . . . . . . . . . . . . . . . . . . . . . . . . 5

  **Admissions** . . . . . . . . . . . . . . . . . . . . . . . . . . . . 5

    Symptoms. . . . . . . . . . . . . . . . . . . . . . . . . . . . . 5

    Diagnosis . . . . . . . . . . . . . . . . . . . . . . . . . . . 12

    Insurance . . . . . . . . . . . . . . . . . . . . . . . . . . . 20

**The Curriculum Can Kill You**. . . . . . . . . . . . . . . . 29

  **Required Courses and Professors**. . . . . . . . . . . 29

    Doctors and Nurses . . . . . . . . . . . . . . . . . . . 29

    Surgeries. . . . . . . . . . . . . . . . . . . . . . . . . . . 31

    Treatments . . . . . . . . . . . . . . . . . . . . . . . . . 43

    Recovery and Therapy . . . . . . . . . . . . . . . . . 54

**The Education Is Priceless**. . . . . . . . . . . . . . . . . . 65

  **Observations and Realities**. . . . . . . . . . . . . . . . 65

    Relationships. . . . . . . . . . . . . . . . . . . . . . . . 65

    Prayers and Blessings. . . . . . . . . . . . . . . . . . 72

Lessons and Reflections . . . . . . . . . . . . . . . . . 79
Graduation . . . . . . . . . . . . . . . . . . . . . . . . . . 85

**Acknowledgments** . . . . . . . . . . . . . . . . . . . . . . . . 89

**About the Author** . . . . . . . . . . . . . . . . . . . . . . . . 91
Connect with Me . . . . . . . . . . . . . . . . . . . . . . . 92

**Proceeds from the University of Cancer** . . . . . . . . . . 93

# PREFACE

*THE UNIVERSITY OF CANCER* CAME to fruition as a result of my son's cancer and then with my own. I would journal during my five-hour treatments of chemotherapy and the long drives to and from my home in San Clemente and USC Keck Medical Center in Los Angeles.

At first, I wondered "why my son" and then soon "why me." I discovered a tremendous new knowledge of how our medical system and insurance system worked. I came to the realization that my care and my coverage was going to require a lot of effort on my part. The insurance system is not an easy labyrinth to navigate. Especially when you're sick with a potentially life-threatening disease. The whole process required new learning and understanding along with a determined persistence and a whole lot of patience.

I also learned a lot about the medical profession and those who work in it. There are a few talented and qualified physicians, in addition to as some who are not so talented or qualified. You'd better figure out which are which; your life depends on it.

I wrote this book to keep my mind sharp while I was dealing with a miserable situation. I wanted to share with other regular people like me who find themselves in a battle with cancer. To all the friends and family members of those with cancer, because I believe them to be the unsung heroes of this experience.

I wrote this book to share my story from an ordinary guy's perspective, to communicate my story with others, and to contribute to others who might benefit from my experience with proceeds that come from the book.

Thank you for your interest in *The University of Cancer*. I pray that through it, I might add some value to your journey.

Blessings,

James Perry

# INTRODUCTION

Each of us has a story to share. Our stories include all our experiences and all the people who have been part of our lives. We all have our broken pieces, emotionally, spiritually, and physically. No one makes it through life unscathed and unscarred by the challenges that life deals us. We are all trying to find those beautiful people whose broken pieces fit together with our broken pieces and something whole can come to life.

Certainly, along the pages of our lives, there are people who, for better or for worse, have had a significant influence on us. Like all stories, the pages that make up our lives are not meant just to be written but read and shared with others. Someone has shared their story with you and others have played active roles in your life. While the stories of our lives are still being written, I believe that we should share how our stories have changed and molded us along the way, and how our stories might help, teach, comfort, or inspire others.

My purpose in writing this book is to share my story and experiences dealing with cancer. To encourage and support other cancer patients and the ones they love who are also affected by cancer in so many ways. To share some of my broken pieces and how those pieces somehow came together to create a beautiful mosaic as a result of my time spent at the University of Cancer.

The University of Cancer is a special place that no one intentionally applies to, no one wants a scholarship to, and no one congratulates you after being accepted to such a prestigious institution of higher education. In fact, when a person is first accepted into the University of Cancer, it is a "cage-rattling experience," and not in a good way.

Picture Tweety Bird, the fictional yellow canary, swinging away on his swing, whistling a beautiful song, when suddenly, Sylvester, the Tuxedo cat, comes along and shakes the shit out of his cage. Tweety Bird falls off his perch, his feathers are completely ruffled, and his whole world is suddenly turned upside down. That is the type of cage-rattling experience you get when you first realize that you have been accepted to the University of Cancer.

And, it's not just the person with the cancer; it's his or her whole family and close friends who get to participate in

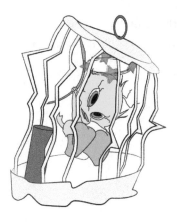

the cage-rattling experience. Their lives too will suddenly be changed; fear and uncertainty will sweep over everyone, and big alligator tears will come pouring out. All of your friends, family, and acquaintances feel sorry for you, and they tell you they will pray for you or offer, "if there is anything I can do for you, just let me know." Of course, there is nothing they can do for you except pray and be available to encourage and support you and your family.

Being accepted to the University of Cancer is the furthest thing from a celebration. Everyone, especially the one accepted, wants to know what he or she did to be honored with such a fine designation. This acceptance causes us to try to understand the symptoms that brought us here in the first place.

On June 5, 2017, my son Julian had the honor of being accepted into the University of Cancer. Five months and four days later, on November 9, 2017, I was accepted to the University of Cancer.

In the pages that follow, I will share my story, experiences, challenges, lessons, and the blessings that come with being accepted into the University of Cancer.

# NO ONE APPLIES

## Admissions

### Symptoms

ON JUNE 5, 2017, I received a call from my son Julian, he told me that he had been diagnosed with cancer and that he would be having surgery the following morning at six A.M. This was a cage-rattling experience for me as a father. Julian and I have a special and close relationship, he is my only son and my best friend. Since Julian was a baby, I've spent a tremendous amount of time with him, cultivating his mind, his confidence, his spirit, his sense of humor, and his playfulness.

I have always had two basic goals in my life, to be a great husband and to be a great father; nothing else really matters to me. When Julian was a young boy, I used to carry him on my shoulders while walking the beach in San Clemente. I would sing the Harry Nilsson lyrics, "People, let me tell you 'bout my best friend, he's a one boy cuddly toy, my up, my down, my pride and joy."

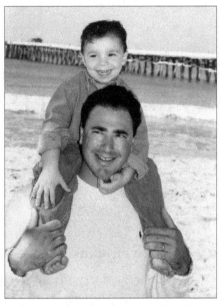

*Julian and me on the beach*
*in San Clemente, California, 1996.*

As a child, I would spend hours watching him ride his bike and his skateboard. When he began playing sports, I coached his baseball teams (we won almost every game). I wanted to teach him to be a winner and that winning was not only fun; winning is important in life. I never missed a baseball practice or game. I never missed a football practice or game. I never missed anything in my son's life, ever.

I drove him all over to visit universities and helped him get accepted to the University of Arizona. I have spent a ton of money supporting my son in anything that he ever wanted to do. I delight in my beloved son. Now, my little boy has cancer! But he is not a little boy anymore; he is twenty-three years old; he had just gotten married in May 2016.

Julian would quickly be admitted to a hospital for surgery to remove his cancer. Once he recovered from the surgery, he would have to endure five hours of chemotherapy each day, five days a week for four weeks. My baby boy was sick, a kind of sickness that does not go away with some medicine, chicken soup, and rest.

All of this happened so fast: one day he was diagnosed, the next day he had surgery, within a couple of weeks, we were moving him back to our home with his new bride Woo Jin. The following week we met with an oncologist to learn about chemotherapy and the treatments that Julian would be enduring over the next few months and what to expect. I watched my twenty-three-year-old son change from a confident, handsome, physically strong young man to a weak, bald, angry, fearful young man. The most heart-wrenching experience I have ever endured.

By mid-September 2017, Julian had already endured a surgery and three weeks of twenty-five hours per week of chemotherapy. Late August and September is a season when kids go back to school, and many people get a cold or the flu. First, my daughter Alexandra caught a cold and worked her way successfully through it. Then Shanna, my bride, worked her way through the flu.

By the end of September, the flu finally got around to me. I could feel it coming on in my throat; my nose was running, I also noticed that my neck was slightly swollen. I went to urgent care to see the doctor. He asked me why I was there. I told him I had the flu and I needed to get rid of it. He told me that I didn't need a doctor for a common cold and to go home, take some cold medicine, get some rest, and eat some chicken soup; the cold would work its way out in a week or so.

I told the doctor that my son Julian was about to begin his fourth week of chemotherapy. Julian had already endured seventy-five hours of chemo and the next week he would endure another twenty-five hours. He was extremely weak, and I did not want any chance of him getting pneumonia from my cold. The doctor understood and gave me some prescription antibiotics and told me I would be fine in a couple days.

The doctor asked if I had any other concerns. I told him that I was concerned with a swollen lump in my neck. The doctor explained that I likely had swollen lymph nodes, which is common with colds. He then said, "If the flu goes away and the lump in your neck doesn't, have it checked." Well, the flu went away, and the lump in my neck did not.

I made an appointment to see my general physician, who I consider a dear friend of over twenty years. Dr. Vincent checked me out, took blood for testing, and suggested that I get an ultrasound scan on my neck to see what he could do to determine the cause of the swollen lymph nodes. I went again to see Dr. Vincent to review the results of the blood test and ultrasound scan. I was a little concerned but not overly concerned. To my delight, my blood work was perfect, and the scan didn't reveal anything resembling cancer.

"What next?" I asked. Dr. Vincent suggested I see an ear, nose, throat (ENT) specialist to get another opinion and made an appointment for me to see a local ENT specialist. I was not able to get in right away; I had a conference I needed to attend out of town in late October. I wasn't able to get an appointment with ENT specialist Dr. Paul in Laguna Hills until November 9, 2017.

While away at the conference in late October, Patrick, a friend of mine and one of our business attorneys, was speaking on compliance. Before he began, he took a moment to share with us how during the last year, in March 2017, he had lost Phil, his law partner of twenty-nine years, to cancer.

He went on to explain that he had lost his wife of thirty-five years in May 2017 to cancer, and that he had lost his thirty-two-year-old daughter to cancer just three months ago in July 2017. It was an emotional announcement and was especially sad when he said that October 25, that exact day, would have been her thirty-third birthday.

Later, I asked him how he managed to get through such a difficult season. Patrick looked at me and said, "Jim, I try not to manage things that are out of my control. It is faith in God and faith alone that has carried me through and continues to carry me today." I shared with Patrick what we had been dealing with about Julian. It was a deep and emotional conversation.

Later that day, Julian called me. I could tell in his voice that he was extremely concerned about what he was about to tell me. As Julian's voice cracked, he told me that his doctors told him that after his surgery and 100 hours of chemotherapy, they believed that his cancer had spread to lymph nodes near his stomach. He told me that this would be a dangerous surgery because the infected lymph nodes were close to and might have grown attached to his inferior vena cava, the major artery that delivered deoxygenated blood from his lower body to his heart. If that artery were severed during surgery, he could bleed to death. If the cancer had attached itself to the artery, he could have cancer in his blood. This was a serious, potentially life-threatening surgery. The doctors who diagnosed it were not qualified or willing to perform the retroperitoneal lymph node dissection surgery. We wept and prayed on the phone together.

When I returned home from the conference, I shared with my friend George what was going on with Julian. George was kind enough to contact a friend of his, Dr. Sinha, a cancer specialist at Keck Medical Center of USC in Los Angeles, to see what he might recommend.

The following week, I was visiting my friend Mr. Bhindi, at his flagship jewelry store in Artesia, California, making plans for a Christmas gift for Shanna. I shared with Mr. Bhindi what was happening with Julian. Bhindi said, "Jim, I have a dear friend and client who is an oncology specialist out of UCLA. If it is OK, I will ask him to see Julian." I readily agreed!

The following day, my mobile phone was ringing. I picked up the call and it was Dr. Sant. He said, "Mr. Perry, this is Dr. Sant; Mr. Bhindi asked me to call you. Tell me about your son." I shared with Dr. Sant what Julian was dealing with. Dr. Sant said, "Get Julian's scan and his records and come to my office tomorrow at eleven A.M., I WILL TAKE CARE OF HIM." Dr. Sant didn't ask what kind of insurance we had, he didn't ask anything about Julian's current doctors, he just said bring him to me and I will take care of him. That is exactly what we did.

We met with Dr. Sant the following day, he examined Julian, gave us his expert diagnosis, and said, "You should have the surgery at Keck Medical Center. I am on staff there and I will personally select your surgeon." Dr. Sant was confident in his diagnosis and assured both Julian and me that he would be cared for by the best physicians in the world, that they would take care of him, and he would make a full and complete recovery. That was the best news we could have hoped for, and that is exactly what he did.

A day or two later, I received a call from Dr. Sinha, who told me that he had known Dr. Sant for over twenty-five years and that together they had made arrangements for Julian to see Dr. Daneshman, one of the finest cancer urologists in the world. With a lot of prayer, meaningful friendships, and relationships, Julian had an appointment with the best and our confidence level rose again.

## Diagnosis

On November 9, 2017, I went to my appointment with ENT specialist Dr. Paul to see what the lump was in my neck. At this time, I felt perfectly fine, the lump in my neck really didn't cause me any discomfort. I have always taken good care of myself with diet, exercise, and mental attitude. I have always been in the gym; I work out with a boxing coach three times each week, weight train three times each week, practice yoga, and walk five miles on the beach every Sunday.

I had absolutely no idea that I had cancer. I felt great. I was happy, confident, my mind was sharp, and I was fit as any fifty-three-year-old man could be. No one in my family or my wife's family had ever had cancer. I felt like I was the most unlikely person in the world to ever develop cancer. But, so was Julian; he was perfectly fit and healthy, but he developed cancer, and he was only twenty-three years old. None of this has any rhyme or reason, a perfectly healthy twenty-three-year-old young man and a perfectly healthy fifty-three-year old man somehow have cancer. Cancer doesn't care what you eat, how much you exercise, how well you cultivate your mind or spirit. Cancer can and will attack anyone at any time.

When I met Dr. Paul for the first time, I had a comfortable and confident feeling that I was with a unique and competent physician. What was unique was that he was a regular guy, and he seemed to actually care about his patients. Additionally, it was clear that he was confident in what he was doing. Dr. Paul examined my throat from the outside, feeling the lump, then examined the inside of my mouth with a light and then with his gloved finger.

When Dr. Paul was finished, he looked at me and said, "I am ninety-five percent certain that you have cancer in your tonsil, and it has spread to your neck." I was shocked! I began to feel hot flashes and disorientation. Dr. Paul asked if I was all right, and I asked for some water. When I came back to consciousness, Dr. Paul was standing in front of me, watching over me. I asked about the water and he said to wait a few moments. He told me that I had fainted. He blew cool air on me as I came back to clear consciousness.

Finally, as I had my bearings back, he gave me the water and we talked. He assured me that I would get through this; that the best thing to do was to get a positron emission tomography (PET) scan and a biopsy. If he was correct, he would remove my tonsil and probably some infected lymph nodes in my neck.

He told me that I would most likely have radiation treatment for five to six weeks after I recovered from the surgery.

As I gathered my thoughts and composure, we spoke more about what he believed I was dealing with. I asked how often he was seeing this type of cancer. He said it was three to four times each month, which was surprising to me. He assured me again that I would get through this and make a 100 percent recovery. I was thankful for his candor, his confidence, and his reassurance. Still, when he asked me my thoughts about his diagnosis and plan for treatment, I replied thank you, but I was 95 percent certain that I was going to see somebody else.

After my cage-rattling experience with Dr. Paul, I was faced with the pleasure of telling the news to my bride Shanna, my daughter Alexandra, Julian, and my staff. I am still in shock from what the doctor just told me. I tried to understand what I did to cause this cancer. Why me? Why my son? How will Shanna and Alexandra respond? Will my business survive? I had a lot of things running through my mind as I traveled the longest, most silent, two-mile drive I have ever been on. I prayed the whole way (with my eyes open). I remember talking to God and asking him, "What did I do to deserve this? What lesson are you trying to teach me? How is it that I am to count this pure joy?"

When I arrived at my office, I parked and made the long silent walk to the building, up the elevator, and into my office.

Everyone asked how it went. I suggested that we meet later in the conference room, as we do every morning. I was able to speak with my daughter Alexandra in her office privately before sharing with the team. I shared with Alexandra what the doctor had to say, we prayed, and she asked, "Have you told Mom?" I had not told her yet; Alexandra was the first to know.

Alexandra is an emotionally mature twenty-year-old young lady. She has composure and grace that is not common in anyone, much less a twenty-year-old girl whose brother was diagnosed with cancer five months ago, endured surgery, and just completed 100 hours of chemotherapy the week before. Now her Popa has cancer. When Alexandra was young, she battled (and continues to battle today) immune thrombocytopenic purpura (ITP), low blood platelets. As a young girl, she had spent a lot of time in the Hematology Department at Children's Hospital of Orange County.

Alexandra grew into a resilient and emotionally tough girl at a very young age and now she would be tested again. In a lot of ways, Alexandra was able to keep a steadfast and positive attitude through a challenging time in our family. I am so thankful that Shanna had Alexandra to lean on, and I am thankful that my daughter had the emotional strength to support and encourage her mom through a challenging season.

Our team met in the conference room, and we went down our list of business, as usual. When we were finished, I shared with them the news that I had been diagnosed with cancer in my tonsil, which had already spread to the lymph nodes in my neck. We prayed together, and they encouraged me. I have the greatest team of bright, talented, caring people ever assembled in a small company; I love them, and they love me. They assured me that I would be all right and that they would run the business exceptionally while I did whatever was necessary to get better.

Then Yadira exclaimed, "Call George's friend!"

Rudy said, "George's friend is an ENT cancer specialist."

George is a client of ours and a dear friend. Yadira ran to her office and wrote Dr. Sinha's number on a pink sticky note and handed it to me. I remembered speaking with Dr. Sinha regarding Julian, but I didn't remember that his specialty was head and neck cancer.

I called Dr. Sinha on his cell phone. When he picked up my call, I said, "Dr. Sinha, this is Jim Perry calling." Dr. Sinha politely interrupted me and said that he had already spoken with Dr. Sant and Dr. Daneshman, and that Julian was in the hands of the best physicians for his surgery to remove the lymph nodes from his stomach. I thanked Dr. Sinha and said, "I am calling about me." Dr. Sinha asked me what was going on.

I told Dr. Sinha that I visited an ENT specialist and that he looked in my mouth with a light, felt around the lump in my neck, stuck his finger in my throat, and told me that he was 95 percent certain that I had cancer in my tonsil and it had spread to my neck. Dr. Sinha said, "Get me a copy of your PET scan, a copy of that doctor's report, and come to my office. I WILL TAKE CARE OF YOU." Just hearing him say those words set me at ease. I believed him, and I knew that somehow, I had the best physician to help me get through this.

Calling my Bride was next, and I prayed for wisdom, peace, and self-control before I dialed the phone. Shanna, like Alexandra, had been dealing with her son Julian and his cancer diagnosis, now she was going to find out that her husband has cancer.

When Shanna picked up the phone, I said, "Hi, darlin'." Shanna asked, "How did it go with the ENT doctor?"

I said, "He claims that he is ninety-five percent sure that I have cancer in my tonsil, and it has gotten into my neck." I told her that I was 95 percent sure that I was going to USC to see Dr. Sinha. Shanna is one tough chick! She dealt with Alexandra as a child with her hematology ITP issues, visiting the hospital two and three time each week. She had been dealing with Julian and his cancer experience since June 5. Now it was November 9, and her husband was calling to tell her that the doctor said he has cancer too.

Surprisingly, Shanna calmly said, "OK, don't worry, we will get through this."

I was shocked, but at this season in our lives, nothing was going to shock my Shanna Lou. Candidly and selfishly, I admit, I was a little disappointed in her response. When Julian told her his news, she had to pull over in her car and cry her eyes out. With me, "Don't worry, we will get through this"? Not one tear! No pulling over her car or even sitting down, just steadfast faith and confidence, UNBELIEVABLE!

Next, my call to my son Julian. No fun. He too is one emotionally, spiritually, mentally tough young man. Julian had been dealing with his own cancer for the last few months. He had told us many times that as miserable as an experience that his cancer was, he would rather endure it than have any of us have to go through the same pain. Julian was confident that we would get through this season together, that we would encourage one another, and even have a competition in beating this thing. We are both competitive, this would just be another challenge that we would have to win. Option B was not an option. He said, "Pop, we will get through this," and we wept together on the phone and prayed some more.

After that, I called my mom and my brothers, Tony and Joe. I don't think any of them thought I was telling them the truth, as each of them were more calm and more confident than I had expected. Or maybe they were just in shock and didn't know what to say or how to react. No one in either Shanna's family or my family had ever had cancer, now both Julian and I were in the battle. I called my best friend Eric in Florida and shared with him the news. Eric was ready to get on a private jet and fly across the country at a moment's notice to be with me and my family.

Friends like Eric are few and far between. I thank God to have such a friend but flying across the country was not necessary and wasn't going to change anything for now.

The whole process of letting family and friends know was a difficult and humbling experience. Their reactions were much the same. I understood that each of them cared, just some more and differently than others. At first, everyone says they will pray for you or they say, "If there is anything I can do, please don't hesitate to call." Then a few weeks later, you never hear from them.

Sharing with loved ones, friends, and family can sometimes be difficult. Many cancer patients choose not to share with anyone outside their immediate family. I felt that way when Julian was first diagnosed. Part of the sharing feels like you don't want to burden others with your problems. There are feelings of failure and disappointment and you don't want to let others down. Some feel just like weeping and going into a hole and hiding, I understand each of those feelings; I felt them all.

I remember talking with Shanna a week or so after Julian's diagnosis, specifically about this idea of letting other people know. We decided to let everyone who cared to know, know.

We felt that we would take all the prayers we could get, that if prayer works, and it does, we wanted as much as we could get. We also learned that because we shared, we found that we were not alone and that many people have been through what we were going through and they shared how they dealt with it.

Some of our friends and clients referred us to specialists who ended up treating us. We would never have met any of the specialists who treated us had we not shared. No one would have known how they could help had we not shared, and thankfully, because we did, they did. I would encourage anyone dealing with cancer to open up and share with as many people as they can. You never know who knows who or what they might know that might make all the difference in the world.

## Insurance

Through Julian's experience, I realized that there was a huge difference between "adequate care" and the "best care." I, like many people, had a lot of "blind faith" in the medical industry. I thought that doctors were special people, that hospitals, nurses, and everyone else involved in the healthcare world had my best interests in mind. Nothing could be further from the truth.

Reflecting on this truth, I am somewhat disappointed that I was so naïve. I have always taught my family and my staff that you can either take what you get, or you can get what you want. Why would I ever consider settling for taking what I get when it comes to my healthcare and the healthcare of my family?

After my diagnosis, my conversation with Dr. Sinha, and especially after Julian's experience with his doctors, I was determined to get the best care. I contacted Dr. Vincent and requested that he refer me to Dr. Sinha, which he was more than willing to do. I also contacted Dr. Paul, who had diagnosed my cancer, and asked that he refer me to Dr. Sinha, which he also agreed to do.

I remember going to the LA Lakers game that evening with my friend George. While waiting to meet George, Dr. Paul was kind enough to call me three or four times to assure me that I would get through this and that he would refer me to Dr. Sinha if that was what I wanted. I told him that I believed Dr. Sinha to be the best doctor in the world to care for the issues that I was dealing with. He agreed that Dr. Sinha was indeed one of the best head and neck cancer specialists in the world.

In fact, Dr. Sinha had been a professor of Dr. Paul while in medical school, but Dr. Paul warned me that I might have to fight with the insurance company to go to him, because Dr. Sinha was what insurance providers consider "out of group." I said, "I am up for the fight." This cancer stuff is some serious shit! Dr. Paul was understanding, and I thanked him for his care and concern for me. In the interim, he suggested that I go through with the PET scan, which he had ordered, as Dr. Sinha would also require one. I agreed.

I made an appointment to have the PET scan done. When I went there, I met a nice enough guy who put me in a dark cold room, stuck a needle in my arm, and injected some stuff that makes the cancer show up on the PET scan. He left me in the dark cold room with some blankets and told me to relax and that he would be back in about forty minutes. I can tell you for certain that there is nothing more relaxing than having cancer stuff pumped into your veins, then being placed in a cold dark room for forty minutes.

When he returned, he took me into another room with a giant tube, he told me to lie on the table in front of the tube and told me that he was going to go behind the glass to the secret place where they operate the PET scan machine. The scan would take about fifteen to twenty minutes. After going in and out of the tube the radiation technician returned and told me the scan was complete. Seemed easy enough.

I mentioned that he must make a ton of money as a radiologist, and he told me that he was just a technician and didn't actually make a ton of money. Then I asked him, "With all the research, all the financial resources, and all the brilliant minds who have been studying and treating cancer for all these years, why haven't they found a cure?"

He looked at the door to confirm that it was still closed, looked at me, and said, "There is no money in a cure; there is big money in treatment." That was encouraging, NOT. I asked him how much this PET scan cost. He said it was about 8,500 bucks! I asked how many scans he does every day, he replied eight to ten PET scans each day. That's about $80,000 every day of the week, fifty-two weeks each year!

I received a call from my insurance company a day or two later and they informed me that I was to see another ENT at Mission Hospital in Mission Viejo. I told the insurance lady that both Dr. Vincent and Dr. Paul had already referred me to Dr. Sinha at USC. She told me that Dr. Sinha was "out of group" and that I had to see a doctor that was "in group."

A week later, Shanna and I visited another ENT doctor in Mission Viejo. He looked in my mouth and felt my neck and agreed with Dr. Paul's diagnosis, then stuck a long scope up my nose, which did a U-turn down my throat where we watched on a TV what he was showing us that he said was cancer. He suggested that I might not have to have surgery and that he could probably just treat me with radiation. I told him that I wanted him to refer me to Dr. Sinha at USC.

The doctor told me that my insurance company would likely not allow me to go out of group, and that he didn't really think I needed to see a specialist like Dr. Sinha. I told him thanks for his opinion and again asked him to refer me to Dr. Sinha. Again, he tried to discourage from requesting a referral.

I asked him, "Do you know who Dr. Sinha is?"

He replied, "Mr. Perry, probably every ear, nose, and throat physician in the world knows who Dr. Sinha is."

So I asked, "How many ear, nose, and throat doctors know who you are?" Then I looked him right in the eye and told him to refer me to Dr. Sinha, and I would deal with the insurance company. I remember thinking to myself that there was no way I was going to let this clown treat me. Finally, he agreed.

Shanna and I went to see Dr. Sinha at USC, where he had reviewed my scan, blood tests, etc., and recommended robotic surgery to remove the cancer in my tonsil and neck surgery to remove the cancer that had moved into the lymph nodes in my neck. I told Dr. Sinha that my general doctor and two ENTs had referred me to see him specifically and that the insurance company was still jacking me around. Dr. Sinha told me that I must fight harder. I have cancer in my head and neck, that this was some serious shit, and that I should insist on seeing him. I asked Dr. Sinha to e-mail his diagnosis and recommendations for treatment so that I would have something meaningful to tell the insurance company.

Dr. Sinha sent me his diagnosis and his treatment plan of (1) surgeon with experience in transoral robotic surgery

(TORS) since 2010; (2) Radiation Therapy Oncology Group (RTOG) clinical trial at Keck Medical Center: TORS and Radiation vs. Chemoradiation Therapy for tonsillar cancer; and (3) speech and swallow rehab during radiation. He also sent about a dozen articles that he had written on the subject that had been featured in medical publications all over the world.

Dr Sinha told me that I must insist on a specialist who has experience performing this specific surgery since 2010.

I asked, "Why since 2010?"

He replied, "There is only one person in the world who has been performing this specific robotic surgery since 2010." Then he smiled. I attempted to read the medical journal articles and quickly realized that this stuff was way over my head, but I knew that Dr. Sinha was the best man for the job, and I had the necessary tools to battle with the insurance company.

By this time, it was early December, and I was assigned to what insurance companies call a "case manager." She was actually very nice and said she would do her best to get the insurance company to allow me to see Dr. Sinha. Also, at this point, I was considering just paying for this surgery and treatment out of my pocket, no matter what the cost. My life was at risk!

A week or so later, I received a call from the case manager; she informed me that the insurance company wanted me to see another ENT specialist at UCI Medical Center. I said to her,

"Look lady, my general physician referred me to Dr. Sinha, as did the two ENTs who the insurance company sent me to." I told her that I had a growing cancer in my head and neck. It was not going away and that if the insurance company did not approve moving me to Dr. Sinha that I would file a lawsuit against the insurance company as they were putting my life at risk with all these delays.

I assured her that if the transfer to Dr. Sinha was not approved in the next day or two that the next call she would receive would be from my attorney. When I hung up the phone, I thought, *I can't afford to get in a legal battle with a giant insurance company.* I might have let my alligator mouth overload my hummingbird brain. The following day she called me and stated, "Mr. Perry, your referral to Dr. Sinha has been approved." It worked! What a battle.

Finally, I called Dr. Sinha's office and told them the news. He called me an hour later and gave me two or three dates to schedule the surgery. After seeing my general physician and two head and neck specialists and battling the insurance company, my surgery was on. I was now going to have cancer surgery followed by chemotherapy and radiation treatment. The real battle was about to begin. Reality set in; for the first time I was really concerned for my family, my business, and my life.

I am a leader; God made me that way. Now my ability to lead was in jeopardy; my true ability to lead would soon be exposed. I am the "rainmaker" at my business, I am the guy who brings in the investment opportunities and the capital to fund them. Without me doing that, we would have no new business. How long could my business survive without me? How well would my team stay together with this type of adversity? How many of them would jump ship and seek greener pastures with more secure employment opportunities? How long would my recurring revenue streams be able to carry the overhead?

These are concerns that business owners face when this type of crisis comes their way. In 2012, President Barack Obama said, "If you've got a business—you didn't build that. Somebody else made that happen." I was wondering who that somebody else was and wondering if that "somebody else" would come along and run the business for me—take all the responsibility, make the rent payment, pay the payroll, the insurance, the taxes, the marketing and advertisement bills, all the supplies required, and manage all the problems in my absence.

I wondered if this "somebody else" that Obama said built this business for me would bring investment opportunities and the capital to fund them so that all the bills, payroll, rent, et cetera, would be taken care of. Not likely. This crisis would certainly challenge my business, as it would any other small business where the leader is sidelined for a period of time.

How would my family get along without me as a husband and father, as a hunter, gatherer, provider, and protector? My bride Shanna was already dealing with her son who had cancer, a new daughter-in-law who was clearly challenged with the circumstances, and a daughter concerned about her brother and now her father.

Families need leadership, they were designed to have mothers and fathers, sons and daughters, each with specific roles and contributions to the whole. Each would have to pick up the pieces and share in the responsibilities of the others. So many times, families crumble apart or abandon ship during these difficult and challenging times.

It can be understandable—so many of us simply don't want to be a burden on our loved ones, so it can seem like the best thing to do is just get out. How would my bride respond? Many marriages crumble in this type of adversity; that is understandable too. Life is tough and getting tougher. There were many times that I wanted to go jump in front of a train, thinking it would make their lives easier. This type of adversity would clearly challenge my family as it does every other family that gets admitted to the University of Cancer.

# THE CURRICULUM
# CAN KILL YOU

## Required Courses and Professors

### Doctors and Nurses

GENERALLY SPEAKING, IN AMERICA AND probably all over the world, when a person has a title of doctor, or there is an MD following his or her name, for some reason we believe that they are highly qualified physicians who can and should be trusted with our health and wellness, even our lives. Unfortunately, nothing could be further from the truth. As in all professions and all aspects of life, there are the exceptional, the adequate, and the incompetent. It happens with politicians, lawyers, accountants, fathers, mothers, landscape maintenance people, pastors, you name it. Doctors and nurses are no different; there are the exceptional, the adequate, and the incompetent.

During my battle with cancer, I had experienced a wide range of care providers and facilities, beginning with my general doctor. As much as Dr. Vincent cared for me and as much as I trusted him, he was clear with me that he was not the guy to treat what I was dealing with. He assured me that I needed a head and neck specialist to help me with my ailment.

I was thankful for his candor and recommendation in addition to his humility in explaining that he was not the best guy for the job. I guess that would make put him in the exceptional category, as he knew his limitations and guided me to more qualified people who could help me.

Dr. Paul was probably qualified to treat me, and I would have trusted him to do so, had I not been able to get to Dr. Sinha. I appreciated Dr. Paul's willingness to refer me to the best. I knew when I asked the so-called "specialist" at Mission Hospital if he knew who Dr. Sinha was, and he told me that every head and neck specialist in the world knew who Dr. Sinha was, and that I didn't need that "advanced specialist." In fact, he was reluctant to refer me, so he sure as hell was not going to be my doctor. I had no confidence in this clown at all! He wasn't even concerned that I received the very best care. I guess, I would define him as probably adequate, most likely incompetent, but clearly not exceptional. What kind of a doctor wouldn't encourage his patient to seek the very best treatment? He really pissed me off.

When I met with Dr. Sinha, he assured me that he would take care of me. Dr. Sinha was exceptionally confident. He had with him two Chinese doctors who were paying close attention to everything Dr. Sinha said and did. These doctors had come a long way to hang out with and learn from him.

Dr. Sinha explained to them how the robotic surgery worked and why it was the best possible procedure to help me with my cancer with the least invasive surgery and the least painful recovery process. Dr. Sinha told me that five years from now, he wanted me to be as healthy and normal as I have ever been. I asked him how long the recovery from the surgery and treatments would take. He replied six months to a year, and he suggested that I plan on one year. He also told me that my success in winning this battle would be 1 percent him and his skills and 99 percent me.

Dr. Sinha was adamant about my responsibility in my own recovery. The success of most of this procedure was going to be up to me, how I managed my mind, my emotions, my spirit, and my physical recovery, including speech and swallow therapy, physical therapy, and my own exercise regimen. I like being held responsible and I think that had a lot to do with my confidence in Dr. Sinha. He would do his best in his part of the process, and it was up to me to do my best. Together, we could achieve the best results.

## Surgeries

My surgery was scheduled for January 2, 2018, at six A.M. I was to be there an hour early at five A.M. Shanna,

Alexandra, and I went to Los Angeles and checked into a hotel room so that we would be close to the hospital the following morning. None of us wanted to get up at 3:30 A.M. to drive ninety miles to the hospital from San Clemente. What a way to spend New Year's Day— 2018 was going to be a new year all right and not in a good way.

The night we stayed in Los Angeles, January 1, there was a huge Rose Bowl game between the Oklahoma Sooners and the Georgia Bulldogs. We had a light dinner and watched the game on TV and went to bed early, hoping to get some sleep before the big day. Oklahoma lost. The hotel was filled with both Sooners fans and Bulldogs fans.

While Georgia fans were celebrating and partying, the Oklahoma fans were in the room directly next to us screaming and hollering at each other so much that security had to step in and tell them to quiet down or they would be removed from the hotel. None of us got any sleep and soon it was four A.M. and time to get up and head to the hospital.

We arrived at the hospital on time, filled out a bunch of paperwork, and went to the surgery center for preparation. I was introduced to all kinds of nurses and doctors, each with a specific role and skill set. These people are exceptional and efficient at what they do; everything was systematic. The place was full, and patients were being processed and prepped for surgery, pretty impressive, really.

They all asked me the same questions over and over again. Finally, Dr. Sinha showed up. I asked him again if he knew what the hell he was doing. He smiled confidently at time and assured me that I was in good hands. I was as ready as I was ever going to be, I guess. I wasn't really scared; I didn't really know what I was in for. I had never had a serious surgery before in my life. It was time for Shanna and Alexandra to leave and time for me to say hello to the anesthesiologist.

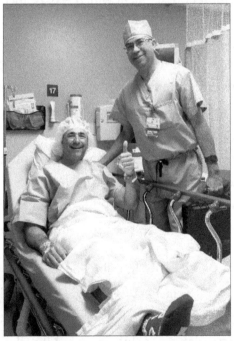

*5:30 A.M., January 2, 2018.*
*All smiles before my surgery.*

Shanna and Alexandra prayed along with all the doctors and nurses, then they both kissed me goodbye. The time had come, and I was now completely in the hands of someone else. There was nothing I could do to help myself. I had to trust these doctors and nurses and trust in the Lord.

My surgery consisted of transoral robotic surgery to remove the left tonsil with a five-centimeter cancer tumor, a chunk of my tongue from inside my mouth, and then cut me from behind my left ear underneath my neck to my chin and removed thirty-one lymph nodes, one of which was a cancerous tumor 5.5-centimeters large.

I had what I was told was a "successful surgery." I was placed in the care of intensive care recovery nurses. My first nurse after surgery comforted me, cared for me, and never left my side. I can assure you that I was not the most pleasant post-surgery patient in the hospital. I wish I could remember her name; she deserves special acknowledgment and thanks. I do remember that she was big, black, and she had yellow eyes. I was not easy on her, but I was sure thankful for her.

After that first long night following surgery, I was sent to a recovery room for the next five days. I had mostly adequate nurses; they did their best to keep me comfortable and alive. I had one particular night shift nurse—I'll call "Fish-Breath Freddie"—who simply wanted to give me narcotics to put me to sleep so he didn't have to deal with me. He not only had the worst bad breath in the history of bad breath, he clearly didn't care and simply provided the absolute minimum effort

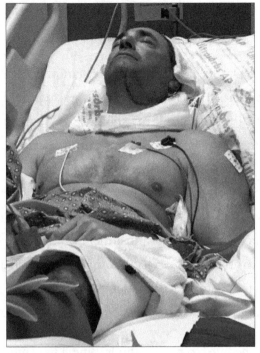

*Recovering from surgery.*
*Not smiling anymore.*

for the people under his care, or at least me. Adequate would be an overstatement at best. In my opinion, this guy was incompetent! I'm not judging; I'm just saying, he was lousy! And his breath was unbelievably bad. This guy could kill a dragon with his breath.

After my surgery and a six-or seven- week recovery from that, I met with Dr. Sinha for a follow- up appointment. He said that he was confident that he had gotten all the cancer, and that he was sending me to see Dr. Bing, a medical oncologist, and Dr. Adam, a radiation oncologist. Both were head and neck cancer specialists.

I asked Dr. Sinha why I needed chemotherapy and radiation treatment, if he thought he had gotten all the cancer. Sinha put his arm around my shoulder and explained to me in otolaryngology, head, and neck cancer specialist language that I couldn't comprehend the purpose of the treatments. What I interpreted was that he had gotten Saddam Hussein out of my tonsil and Osama bin Laden out of my neck, and that the chemo and radiation treatment would make sure there were no terrorist sleeper cells that might sneak up and try to kill me. I understood this analogy better than his technical explanation, but at least we were on the same page.

I was scheduled to meet with Dr. Bing. I remember sitting in the medical oncology room with my nurse Sophia, an exceptional nurse. She asked me a bunch of questions, did some tests—my blood pressure, the routine stuff—and told me that Dr. Bing would be in to see me. A few minutes later, a little Chinese lady popped into my room and introduced herself as medical oncologist Dr. Bing. I was shocked! This lady looked to me like a sixteen-year old, 100-pound, Chinese high school student that I could snap in two if necessary. Turned out she was actually a thirty-one-year old head and neck oncology specialist.

Dr. Bing asked me a bunch of questions, and she seemed confident to me. I shared with her what I had been through, what I was dealing with, my background, and my experience with my son Julian and his cancer. She actually seemed interested in me, which was both weird and refreshing, as she must have had hundreds of poor shmucks like me to deal with.

I asked her about her family. She shared that she had a one-year-old little boy and that her husband was still back in Connecticut completing his education. I asked her where she went to school, and she said that she also had gone to school in Connecticut.

I asked her, "Did you go to UConn? They have a great women's basketball program." She humbly said, "No." She told me that she had graduated from Yale University!

I asked, "Why not Harvard?"

She confidently said, "Yale has the best head and neck cancer oncology school in the world." She graduated at the top of her class. WOW! This chick was smart!

I asked her why in the world would she choose a profession in cancer with all the pain, grief, illness, and all the negative stuff that comes with being in the cancer business. Clearly a young lady as smart as she was could have chosen a much easier and less stressful profession, which would pay her a ton of money.

She told me that science and biology came easy to her, that she had friends or family members who had dealt with cancer, and that she wanted to help people like me. I was shocked again!

I asked her, "Can you cure cancer?"

She looked at me and without hesitation said, "I can cure your cancer, Mr. Perry."

Shocked for the third time in twenty minutes, I lay back on the bed and thought, *Thank you, Jesus! I have an exceptional medical oncologist who is confident that she can cure my cancer.*

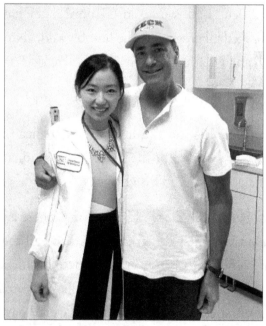

*Dr. Bing, medical oncologist extraordinaire.*

Next, I went to meet Dr. Adam, head and neck radiation oncology specialist at USC Norris Comprehensive Cancer

Center. When I checked in at the front desk, they told me to take the elevator to the basement where the radiology department was. I went to the basement. The elevator door opened; there were no windows, everything was gray, radiation signs everywhere.

I thought, *this must be the dungeon where people come to be tortured.* I figured out how to get to the lobby, where at least there was a waiting room with windows, even a sliding glass door that went outside to a lower level of the campus. I was somewhat relieved.

Soon I was escorted into a room by a nurse. There were more of the same questions that it seemed like I had answered a hundred times before. I was told to wait. There is a lot of waiting going on when you have cancer; you have to be "patient" when you are a cancer patient.

Soon the door opened, and this thirty-something-year-old handsome Italian-looking guy walked in and introduced himself as Dr. Adam, head and neck radiation oncologist. I remember thinking, *Who are all these young people? Shouldn't they be older and wiser looking?* I guess at fifty-four years old, Marcus Welby, M.D., has long since retired and there are new younger smarter physicians running the place now.

Dr. Adam and I got along well. He was confident in the treatment that Dr. Sinha and Dr. Bing were providing and

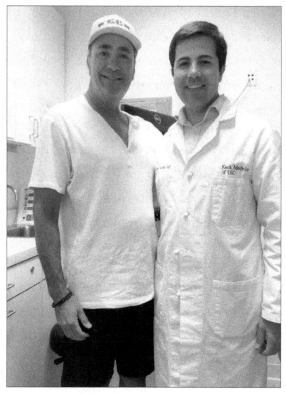

*Dr. Adam, radiation oncologist*
*extraordinaire.*

that the radiation treatment they had prescribed would do the trick. He shared with me what I should expect, encouraged me to continue working out and eating as much as possible because a fit and well-nourished body would be beneficial for what I was going to go through. Seemed easy enough to me, after watching Julian go through the chemotherapy treatment that he went through, radiation seemed like a piece of pie. Boy was I wrong!

I made an appointment to be fitted for my "mask." I remember meeting a couple of radiation technicians, Mike and Chris, who were going to help me with the making of my mask and a special mouthpiece that was required. They told me to take off my shirt and lay on a metal table. Then they stuck some gummy stuff in my mouth, told me to bite down and hold it there.

Next, they brought this plastic mesh-looking sheet with a metal frame around most of it and did some measurements. Mike went into the "secret room"—something like where the Wizard of Oz would go. Chris took the mesh sheet and soaked it in some really hot water.

He told me to stay still and then snapped the mesh sheet on the table I was lying on, as the plastic mesh molded around my head, neck, and chest. He began to dig a hole where my mouth was, and soon the mesh screen had hardened. They unbolted me from the table, took the hardened gummy stuff out of my mouth, told me I was finished, and they would see me in a week or so.

I asked Chris to show me the mask, which he did. I thought it was kind of cool. I asked him to take a picture of me with it on. I asked Chris if I could keep this thing when I was finished with the treatments. He said I could if I wanted to. When I asked him if other patients wanted to keep their masks, he said some do, while some don't want anything to do with it.

Some wanted to take it home and run over it with their cars. Apparently, these patients didn't think the mask was as cool as I did. Soon enough, I would find out why.

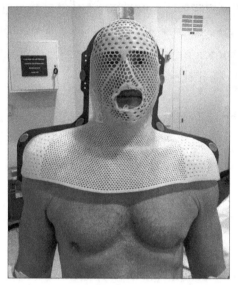

*My new radiation mask.*
*Seemed cool at the time.*

I met with Dr. Adam again to schedule my radiation and chemo treatment. He told me that I would do chemotherapy once each week and radiation every day for seven weeks. I told him that every day would be a challenge, as I live in San Clemente, which is only eighty-five miles one way to USC Norris Comprehensive Cancer Center. With Los Angeles traffic, it could take as long as two to four hours each way.

He suggested that I move closer to USC for the next couple of months. I asked if there was another radiation oncologist who was closer to San Clemente that he could refer me to. He said that there was a doctor at Scripps Memorial Hospital in La Jolla that I could see, but other than that, there were not any head and neck radiation oncologists that he could recommend.

In the interim, my insurance company kept trying to reroute me to a local radiation oncologist, one who was about three miles from my office, certainly a lot more convenient. I asked Dr. Adam if I could see the local radiation oncologist. Dr. Adam said I could, but he would not refer me to anyone who was not a head and neck specialist. I figured that if it was three miles down the road, instead of eighty-five miles one way in LA traffic, that it was worth at least a visit.

I made an appointment with the radiation oncologist at Saddleback Memorial Medical Center. Shanna came with me to meet this guy. He told me to prepare for the worst thing that could ever happen to me, and that this would be the most excruciating experience of my life. I asked a bunch of questions; he did his best to answer.

Shanna and I looked at each other and agreed to get the hell out of there. This was like a meeting with Dr. Kevorkian, the famous doctor of death! The 170-mile round trip to USC every day now seemed perfectly convenient.

### Treatments

I remember being scheduled for chemotherapy first. It was Friday, March 9, 2017. Shanna and I arrived at the treatment center, signed in, and we were showed to our La-Z-Boy chair for the treatment. We expected to begin at 10:30 A.M. About 12:30 P.M., my first treatment began.

I asked the nurse if I was going to get out of there before 4:30 P.M., as we would have a two- or three-hour drive home. She told me that I would be there for seven to eight hours! I wanted to kill her.

I told her, "Look, lady, my son just went through four, week-long sessions of chemotherapy, and his treatments only took four-and-a-half hours each day. Why are mine going to take eight hours?"

She told me, "That's just how long it takes." Great answer.

Just before six o'clock, she moved me to another room, where I met Cynthia, the head chemo treatment nurse.

I asked Cynthia why my treatment takes so long when Julian's treatment only took four hours.

She said, "Some nurses are better and more experienced than others."

I told her that I wanted the best nurse, and I wanted to be in and out in four hours.

Cynthia said that she would take care of me from then on, and that is exactly what she did.

44

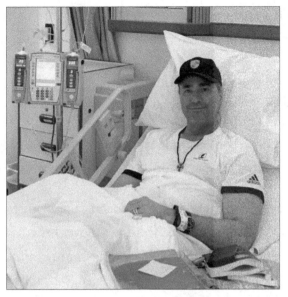

*March 9, 2018, first long day of chemotherapy.*

I was in and out in four to five hours every time from then on. I was able to schedule my chemotherapy treatments at nine A.M. every Friday thereafter with Cynthia, which allowed Shanna and I to get on the road before three P.M. for the two-hour drive home.

The following Monday, I began the radiation treatment. I was apprehensive and somewhat concerned for what I was about to endure. I checked in and was told that someone would be with me shortly. They tell you that a lot in hospitals.

Soon, a door opened, and my name was called. I was escorted into the torture chamber. They told me to put my mouthpiece in, take my shirt off, and lie down on a cold metal table. They told me that they were going to put my mask on and buckle me to the table, and that they would all leave the room and run the radiation machine from the secret room.

I asked if everyone was going to leave.

They said, "Yes, everyone but you. But don't worry, we'll be back in about twenty minutes." Then they left the room.

I was on my back on a cold metal table with my mask on, buckled to the table so I couldn't move. I was scared; so, I began to pray and sing worship songs in my mind. About eight or ten minutes later, the door opened, the radiation techs came back in, unbuckled me from the table, and told me I was finished for the day. WOW, that was easy! I was shocked and glad to get out of there. I would return the following day and every Monday through Friday with both chemotherapy and radiation on Fridays.

During the first three weeks, I would drive by myself Monday through Wednesday. Shanna would come with me on Thursdays, and we would check in to the LA Westin Bonaventure Hotel to stay every Thursday night, this would allow us to be on time for early morning radiation on Friday, blood tests, then chemotherapy. It was not too bad. Those first few weeks, Shanna and I got to stay in a nice place and have dinner together at the top of the hotel, which has a revolving restaurant with the best views in Los Angeles.

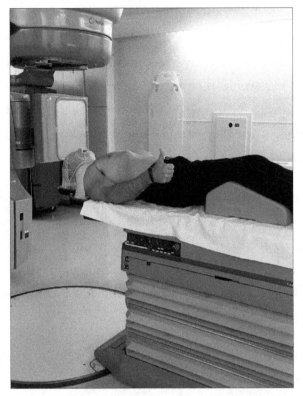

*Radiation torture chamber.*
*The most miserable experience of my life.*

Then week three came along, I had already lost about twenty pounds. I was growing weak and fatigued easily. For the remaining four weeks, someone would have to drive me to and from the hospital for radiation Monday through Wednesday. Every day, it was someone else's turn. Julian and Alexandra would drive me; my dear employees Rudy and Yadira would drive me; even my attorney and dear friend Daniel would drive me. Each of them was so good to me and patient with me.

47

Each of them came with me into the torture chamber and watched as I lay on that cold metal table, while the technicians bolted my mask over my head, neck, and shoulders onto the table. They would then leave and wait for me to come out of the torture chamber, weaker and more scorched from the radiation. Then they would drive me back to the office, so they could return to work.

We had some deep conversations during those rides, and some very quiet ones. As miserable as it was, our relationships grew deep and more meaningful, and I am thankful for that. Shanna continued to drive me on Thursdays, so we could stay all night and be early for radiation and chemotherapy on Friday mornings.

The wonderful time together and enjoying dinner on Thursday nights became less and less wonderful. Soon we would just check into the room, and I would be in bed by four o'clock in the afternoon. I remember one Friday morning during the last couple of weeks of radiation. I was so weak and miserable that when I got up in the morning to go down to the lobby to get coffee for Shanna and me, on the elevator ride down, I shit my pants.

It was humiliating and kind of funny at the same time. I did the march of the penguins to the nearest bathroom, so I could clean up the mess. I did my best, then went out, got the coffee, and returned to the room.

Shanna said, "That took a long time. Was there a line?"

I said, "Oh, there was a line all right, a line of diarrhea, dribbling out of the bottom of my trousers from the elevator all the way to the restroom."

In 1987 when I met Shanna, I fell in love with her beauty (this chick was smoking hot, still is). My love grew for her, as I recognized that there was a purity about her, a gentleness and faithfulness that I had never recognized in anyone before. My mom told me that if I didn't marry Shanna, that someone else would. I wasn't gonna let that happen, so on May 26, 1991, she became my bride.

Shanna has the patience and kindness of a saint. Twenty-seven years prior, when we were married, the pastor asked, "Do you promise to love one another in sickness and in health?" We were young, dumb, and healthy back then, the furthest thing from our minds was cancer, but she would certainly keep up her end of the promise.

On Thursday, April 19, 2018, I completed my last week of treatment. The radiation technicians who had been administering my treatments for the last seven weeks presented me with a diploma certificate for completing the most grueling class they have at the University of Cancer. They have a gong hanging on the wall, that everyone who completes the treatment and earns their diploma gets to bang. They handed me the gavel.

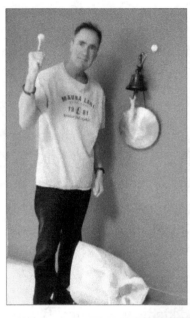

*Final day of radiation
7:19 A.M. treatment.
Bang the gong!*

*Fabulous radiation
technicians who saw me
through the whole process.*

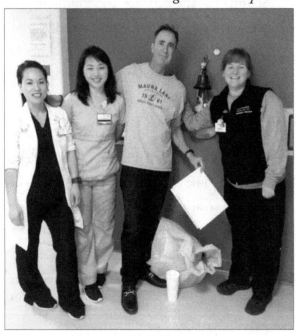

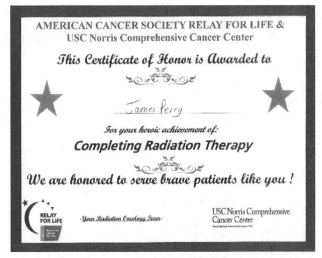

AMERICAN CANCER SOCIETY RELAY FOR LIFE &
USC Norris Comprehensive Cancer Center

*This Certificate of Honor is Awarded to*

*James Perry*

*For your heroic achievement of:*
**Completing Radiation Therapy**

*We are honored to serve brave patients like you !*

RELAY FOR LIFE · *Your Radiation Oncology Team-*    USC Norris Comprehensive Cancer Center

*Received the most difficult diploma*
*I have ever earned.*

When I first began treatment and they told me I would get to bang the gong when I was finished, I was determined to knock that thing off its hinges. Now, I was so weak, that when I finally did get to bang the gong, I could barely make any noise. It was pitiful and sad, but I was finished and hoped to never return. Shanna and I got the hell out of there for what we had hoped would be our last time.

Little did we know, two days later, on Saturday April 21, I was ready to die. Shanna was concerned and was trying to reach my doctors at the hospital, but it was the weekend. I had not eaten anything or had any fluids in five or six days. I had lost over forty-five pounds. I was extremely weak, and my skin was gray, like a dead person.

I was able to help Shanna get Dr. Sinha's phone number from my cell phone. Finally, she was able to reach him and share with him her concerns.

Dr. Sinha asked, "Can you get Jim to the USC medical center?" Shanna said, "Absolutely, we will be there as soon as we can."

About two hours later, we walked into the lobby at Keck Medical Center of USC, and Dr. Sinha was waiting for us in the lobby. I was admitted to the hospital where they began to hydrate me intravenously. After being hydrated for fourteen hours, finally I went to the bathroom and peed. Shanna stayed with me in the hospital that night; it was a long, long night with not much sleep for her.

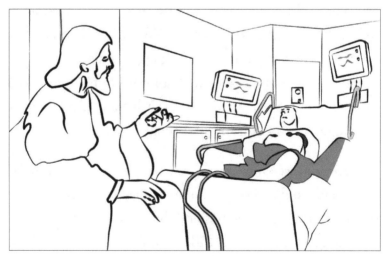

*My vision of Christ appearing at my bedside after my surgery.*
*The ultimate Healer, Comforter, Redeemer, Savior, Friend.*

I remember praying to Jesus and telling Him that I was prepared to go, that I was not afraid and that in fact I was anxiously willing to die. Jesus appeared at my bedside, looked at me, and held out His hand. He said, "James, you have always been in My hands; you are in My hands now; and you will always be in My hands." He then told me, "I am the only One in Heaven, and on earth, and under the earth, who has authority to call you home, not cancer." He said, "I have work for you to do and you have value to add to others and to the kingdom of heaven."

For me, death had lost its sting, there was nothing to be afraid of. As David wrote (Psalm 27:1, NIV), "The Lord is my light and my salvation—whom shall I fear? The Lord is the stronghold of my life—of whom shall I be afraid?"

The next day, Sunday, I was somewhat coherent while they continued to hydrate me and fill me with some sort of nutrition. I was in tremendous pain and could not even swallow my own saliva. I was really miserable. As the day grew on, I continued to get better and encouraged Shanna to go home and get some rest and let the nurses take care for me. She reluctantly agreed, but she was looking forward to a good night's sleep at home in her own bed.

After Shanna left, later that afternoon, the nurse came around as her shift was ending and introduced me to the night shift nurse. To my dreadful surprise, it was Fish-Breath Freddie, the same night nurse I had after my surgery in January. You should have seen the look on their faces when I exclaimed, "Oh, no! Not Freddie. He is the worst!" Freddie claimed he didn't remember me from back in January, but I sure as hell remembered him and the most god-awful breath you can imagine.

It was a long, long night. When Monday morning came, I was feeling much better. The doctors came to check on me. I felt I was good enough to go home. They wanted to make sure that I would eat and drink water to hydrate myself, which I did. About 10:30 A.M., Shanna arrived with Alexandra to see how I was doing and to speak with the doctors about my progress. The doctors told them that as long as I would eat some solid food and drink water, they felt comfortable with sending me home. About one P.M., we were discharged from the hospital again, hopefully for the last time.

## Recovery and Therapy

Before the chemo and radiation treatments, I first had to recover from the surgeries. I vividly remember how painful my neck and trapezius muscles in my shoulders felt. I didn't understand why my upper back and shoulders were in such excruciating pain. The range of motion in my left arm and shoulder was extremely limited. My tonsil was removed, and I couldn't swallow. A chunk of my tongue was sliced off where the cancer had spread. My neck was cut open from behind my ear down my neck and up under my chin to remove the cancer and affected lymph nodes. I was a mess!

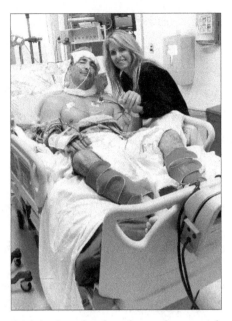

*My darling bride, always by my side.*

When I woke up, Shanna and Alexandra were there praying over me. I was so glad to see them, but I could see fear and concern on their faces. I was exhausted and in deep pain. Nurses came in and seemed to be ever-present with comforting pain medication. There were lots of wires, lights, and beepers that never stopped blinking and making noise.

The doctors came to see how I was doing, but I had no comprehension of what they were saying or doing, I felt like I was just dying or barely surviving, I didn't care which. Shanna and Alexandra were exhausted and once they felt comfortable, they went back to the hotel to get some much-needed rest. It had been a long, long day.

The following morning, Shanna and Alexandra came to see me. I was in deep pain, highly drugged with stuff, and tired. I don't remember much and did my best to get some sleep. Alexandra needed to get home to run our business, and Shanna needed rest. Next, I woke up and recognized my son Julian and his bride Woo Jin in the room.

Julian said, "Hey, Pop."

I said, "You don't look so good. Are you OK?"

Julian said, "I have never seen you like this before."

I looked at Woo Jin and she was weeping. I had never seen her cry; it broke my heart. I felt like I had let them down, and I didn't like that. Julian is a world-class man of prayer, and he prayed over me. I told him and Woo Jin that I would get through this and we would go to Portofino soon. They told me Portofino wasn't going anywhere, it would be there when I got better; just get some rest for now.

I was in that surgery recovery room for five long days. I had needles in my veins, plugs glued to me, drugs pumped into me, and lights and beepers going off constantly. The days were better than the nights. At night, when I was trying to sleep, I was awakened every two hours to check my blood pressure and vital signs.

Fish-Breath Freddie would pump me full of morphine and tell me to go back to sleep. I always felt that he would never listen to me and just wanted to give me some drugs, put me to sleep, and go back to eating stinky food and playing video games on his phone. (I really don't know what he was doing, and he probably was doing a great job.)

It was a long five days. I hadn't eaten anything solid, just soup and Jell-O. One of the doctors came in to see how I was doing, I told her that I was fine, and I wanted to go home. She told me that they wouldn't release me until I could eat some solid food, or else they would put a hole into my stomach and feed me through a tube. I told her to bring me a submarine sandwich and I would eat the whole damn thing, just get me out of there!

Shanna and Alexandra came back to see me, hoping to get me released from the hospital. I ordered some pasta and marinara sauce to eat. The nurses told me that if I could eat the solid food, I could go home. I gobbled up that lousy pasta as fast as I could, so I could get the hell out of there. We were released from the hospital a couple of hours later and drove home to San Clemente.

Recovery from the surgery, as I remember, seemed to go relatively well. For the first few weeks, I could barely eat anything. I couldn't shave; I looked like a malnourished convict. Within five or six weeks, I was back in Dr. Sinha's office for follow-up. Dr. Sinha told me that once I had completed the radiation and chemotherapy treatments, I would have to have lymphedema therapy, speech and swallow therapy, and physical therapy.

My recovery from the chemo and radiation treatments was long and difficult and continues to be difficult even over a year-and-a-half later while I write this. The entire process—the surgeries, the chemotherapy, and the radiation—damn near killed me. There were times when I wanted to die.

Before my surgery, I was fifty-three years old, 193 pounds, with 13 percent body fat, exceptionally strong and fit. I had been lifting weights three days a week, doing yoga twice each week, and boxing twice each week. I was fit. When I came home in April after almost dying of dehydration on April 26, 2017, I weighed 145 pounds; I had lost 48 pounds. I remember looking in the mirror at myself and wanting to cry at what I saw. I was unrecognizable to myself! My hair was gone; none of my clothes fit anymore. It was UGLY! I looked like E.T. the Extra - Terrestrial, and I was extremely weak.

I could barely chew or swallow anything, I remember it taking me forty-five minutes to eat one scrambled egg. I tried to drink protein shakes to get some nutrition in my body and to add some weight. During the first two or three weeks, I slept a lot. About mid-May, I would go for short walks to get some movement, and I began to eat more solid foods.

My taste buds were all screwed up, everything had a metal taste to it, most things tasted like I was eating aluminum foil.

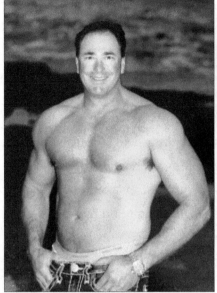 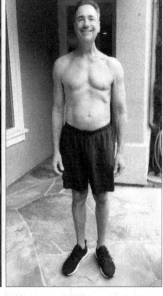

*Before cancer. Summer 2017,*     *After cancer. Summer 2018,*
*195 lbs, strong & fit.*          *140 lbs, weak & frail.*

Anything cold was brutal for me to eat or drink, and anything spicy or hot would make my scalp sweat profusely while the rest of my body from my neck down would be freezing cold and shivering.

My saliva glands were all screwed up too. I had severe dry mouth; I never knew how painful it was to suffer from dry mouth. I would pour this goop in my mouth, swish it around and gargle it, then spit it out to somewhat numb the pain from the dry mouth. My saliva glands had taken a beating and could barely produce enough spit to lubricate any food to get it down my throat. Surprisingly, the dry mouth was one of the worst and most painful aftereffects of the radiation treatment. You never know how valuable your saliva is until you don't have any.

I was scheduled to do speech and swallow therapy with a nice lady named Mara, a speech- language pathologist and occupational rehabilitation specialist. I had to learn how to do all kinds of tongue-strengthening exercises. After the radiation and chemo treatments, my mouth would barely open wide enough to put my finger in. I had to do mouth-opening exercises to increase the range of motion in my jaw, so that my mouth would open wide enough to eat solid food.

I had to relearn how to swallow, without swallowing my tongue. I had electrodes glued to my neck below my mouth to stimulate muscle contractions to strengthen the muscles in my neck and jaw. This went on for months. Mara was a gracious therapist; she explained why we were doing what we were doing and made the whole process as comfortable as possible. I enjoyed meaningful conversations with her about all kinds of different subjects. She is a smart lady with exceptional skill and understanding. I enjoyed working with her a lot.

I also had to have physical therapy and continue to do so today. Dr. Sinha referred me to Kimi at USC. I had lost 80 percent of the range of motion in my left shoulder and arm from nerve damage caused by the surgery. I had lost a tremendous amount of muscle mass from the surgery and all the chemo and radiation treatments. I was weak and had to learn and do difficult and specific exercises to rebuild my range of motion and my strength.

I learned how to use foam rollers to develop flexibility and increase range of motion. I did a lot of exercises on instability balls to engage core muscles and to increase strength and lots of stretching. As I write this, over a year-and-a-half removed from my last chemo treatment, I still have maybe 60 percent of my range of motion back in my left shoulder and arm. It is a long and painful process.

Kimi worked with my boxing coach Frank and my yoga and recovery coach Audri, on specific exercises and movements to maximize my recovery efforts. Frank incorporated specific punching movements and dexterity exercises that we practiced during our boxing sessions. Frank and I also did a lot of rehab exercises with rubber bands and a lot of instability exercises to improve my balance.

Audri is also an expert in physiology, and we worked with specific foam roller movements, stretching and yoga movements, to increase my range of motion and flexibility. I am in the gym doing physical therapy every day of the week, and it is paying off. I weight train two days each week, box two days each week, do yoga two days each week, and walk five miles on the beach every Sunday. All these things are contributing to my full physical recovery, and I enjoy the process. The human body is extremely resilient, and all these physical exercises help tremendously.

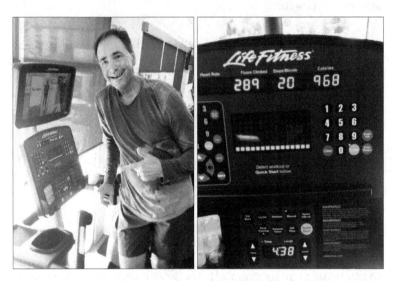

*Summer 2019, 170 lbs.*
*One hour on the stairmill, level 9, 968 calories*
*Climbed 20 steps per minute, 289 floors. Getting fit again*

The physical body is not the only recovery needed. The mind is affected in so many negative ways. Your confidence can leave you, and you can begin to make decisions out of fear and doubt instead of confidence, prudence, and discernment. Depression can come along and dampen your days and your dreams.

Even though my oncologist told me that I was doing well, there were times when a deep, deep sadness would come over me. It would bring tears to my eyes that wouldn't stop.

Posttraumatic stress disorder (PTSD) isn't just for war veterans. Cancer patients experience PTSD and not just physically and mentally, but also spiritually, relationally, and financially as well.

# THE EDUCATION
# IS PRICELESS

## Observations and Realities

### Relationships

ONE OF THE OFTEN-UNAPPRECIATED BENEFITS of cancer is that it accelerates the process of identifying your true friends and loved ones. Most of us have many family members, friends, acquaintances, and associates but are indeed fortunate to have a handful of really true friends. Some relationships with friends and family or even acquaintances are so rich and deep, while others are shallow and superficial or even nonexistent. I have heard it said that people will bring flowers to your funeral, but they won't bring you soup when you're sick, a very accurate statement.

People who you think deeply care about you simply don't, and people who you might have thought didn't care really do.

I'll share just one of the disappointing relationships. Although there are plenty and focus more on the relationships that were so supportive and genuinely caring.

When Julian was diagnosed with cancer, one of the first calls I made was to the "pastor" of our church in San Clemente. Pastor Mark was our neighbor for ten years when we first moved to San Clemente. His son Brandon and Julian have been friends since they were two years old.

In 2016, just one year earlier, Pastor Mark baptized Julian on Easter Sunday. For some foolish reason, we felt that Mark, a "friend, neighbor, and pastor," would show some concern, some gentleness, some compassion, and some comfort, as he had known our family and specifically Julian for over eighteen years.

When I spoke with Mark and told him of Julian's cancer, he was cold and nonchalant; he didn't even offer to pray with me. I was surprised and disappointed. His response hurt my feelings and kind of pissed me off.

I said to myself, "This guy is no pastor. He is an entertainer and not even a good one." I have never been to his church again.

One time I crossed Mark's path in the local grocery store when he saw me and tried to avoid eye contact with me. He had to acknowledge me later when I was standing next to him in line. He asked how Julian was doing. I said that Julian was struggling with the chemo treatments, but his mind and spirit were strong. I then told him that I also had been diagnosed with cancer.

Mark asked about my cancer and the expected treatment and commented, "Wow, you guys have been through a lot."

I haven't spoken to him, seen, or heard from him since. It is disappointing when you are challenged with cancer and people you had hoped would care or show some compassion or empathy simply don't. My "father" never even called me.

Shanna and I have met many "friends" through the years. Many are parents of friends of our kids; we spent a lot of time with these people going to football games, baseball games, and cheer competitions. We had a lot in common it seemed. But when cancer showed up, we had nothing in common anymore, they simply disappeared. What a blessing!

Then there are people who drop everything they are doing to care for you or at least pray and encourage you. Shanna and I visited a new church in San Clemente, a small community church with maybe 200 people who regularly attend. This church, and the head pastors, Ron and Dave, immediately embraced us; we felt accepted and loved. We hadn't even shared with any of them the issues we were dealing with. When we did, they embraced us even more!

Pastor Ron came to my home during my recovery and just sat on the couch, talked with me, and listened to me.

That was encouraging. My staff each took turns driving me to radiation treatments every day and assured me that they would take great care of the business while I dealt with my cancer and the treatments I would have to go through. That's exactly what they did. In fact, they set a record of new business in March of almost eight million dollars in new transactions, and we actually finished 2018 with a record year. Remarkable, considering what we went through.

Another beautiful surprise was all the people at my gym. So many of them were glad to see me back and told me they had been praying for me. I hardly know these people. I only see them about an hour each day at the gym, just friendly hellos and encouragement. But they genuinely cared. I sent a text to my friend Rudy and our yoga instructor Audri when I learned that I was cancer free. When Audri announced to the class the news, the class cheered! WOW! I didn't see that coming.

My friend and attorney Daniel has helped me with legal matters, family estate planning matters, and business succession planning. A few years ago, while helping me with succession planning for my business, Daniel suggested that I purchase a disability insurance policy and overhead-disability insurance policy. I had never even heard of overhead-disability insurance before. He explained that this would cost me five or six thousand bucks each month. I thought he was crazy, but he is my attorney and I pay him to advise me, so I bit the bullet and bought the policies.

When I was diagnosed with the cancer, I spoke with Daniel and he offered to help in any way he could. I asked him if he could help me with the disability insurance claims on the policies that he recommended I should buy. The disability policies turned out to be one of the best business decisions I have ever made. My insurance company, Northwestern Mutual, has exceeded all my expectations. The policy benefits have enabled me and my company to survive the last year and a half without having to concern myself with having enough cashflow to make my payroll and pay my rent. The disability policies I bought from Northwestern Mutual did exactly what they were designed to do—take care of me and my business overhead while I was disabled.

Daniel handled all my disability insurance claims and drove me to my treatments. He never charged me a dime! This guy could charge $750 an hour and spent many, many hours dealing with my insurance company to insure my disability benefits. He told me he was my friend and that he loved me and that there was no way he could charge me for his work.

Daniel is a unique man. He is a successful attorney, has made a ton of money, and he is the kindest and most gentle man I have ever known. Daniel has a nonprofit organization called Rescue Humanity, where he runs two orphanages with over fifty children that he houses, clothes, feeds, and privately educates out of his own pocket. I owe a deep debt of gratitude to Daniel. He is not only a dear friend; he is also a unique and beautiful man. The world could use more men like Daniel.

Eric, my best friend since childhood, lives on the other side of the country in South Florida. I would speak with him regularly on the phone as I was enduring this whole process. Eric always has something positive to say and always makes me laugh. Even when it hurt so bad to laugh, it was great for my soul and spirit to laugh with my friend.

Now that I am cancer free, Eric and I are spending more time together even though we live on opposite ends of the country. Cancer made an already unique and wonderful friendship even deeper and more fun. There is nobody I would rather go to dinner with and laugh so obnoxiously loud that we bother everyone else in the restaurant. Then we would laugh even louder because with our twisted sense of humor, we found that to be funny too. Deep and sincere friendships are few and far between, and a whole lot of laughter is a great healer. Eric is my best friend in the whole wide world; I love and appreciate him dearly.

It is humbling to know there have been so many beautiful and wonderful people who genuinely cared and prayed for me. I am so thankful for each and every one of them. I could write for pages and pages about the beautiful caring people who have touched my life.

Top of the list is my bride Shanna Lou. Shanna and I have been together since the summer of 1987. We have a wonderful son and a beautiful daughter. We have enjoyed many successes and many challenges along the way. In 2017, Shanna was faced with the reality of her son Julian being diagnosed with cancer. Then four months and five days later, her husband was diagnosed with cancer.

The same reality faced my daughter Alexandra—her brother and her pop had cancer. These two beautiful women are tough chicks. They are rocks; they are courageous, loving, patient, and smart. I don't know that I would have desired to fight and live like I did without my need to hunt, gather, provide, and protect my girls.

I remember speaking with Brendette, the receptionist at USC Norris Comprehensive Cancer Center about Shanna and Alexandra. I told her, "You need a strong companion for this part of the ride." Her comment was that not everyone has a strong companion like Shanna Lou. Thank you, darlin', for being my bride. And thank you, Alexandra, for seeing your mom through a difficult season that had to be just as difficult for you.

My daughter-in-law Woo Jin married Julian in May 2016. Woo Jin was born and raised in South Korea. She came to the US to attend UCLA, where she graduated at the top of her class. Julian and Woo Jin are young newlyweds and should be enjoying a honeymoon period, moving to a new home, beginning careers, and starting a family. Instead, Julian was diagnosed with cancer, they had to move from their own home in Los Angeles into our home in San Clemente. Julian had to quit school and Woo Jin had to quit her job.

Somehow, they have made it through the challenges of cancer. No one would volunteer for this set of circumstances, yet she loved Julian and cared for him. I am so thankful that my son has a bride like Woo Jin. She is not only a blessing to him, she is a blessing to our whole family, and we love her deeply.

## Prayers and Blessings

I am the product of a praying mother and praying grandmothers. I have been prayed for by these women since before I was born. I believe in the power of prayer and that the Lord of the universe not only loves to hear our prayers, He answers them and blesses us. He doesn't always answer them the way we are hoping for, and the blessing usually isn't what we were expecting, but He always answers them for our good and for His glory.

I have what I call a satchel of sufficiency of the evidence of the past where prayer and God's blessings worked in my life. These are real-life experiences when I know that God is working in me, through me, and for me, for His glory. Some might call it coincidence or good luck, but I know it to be much deeper than that. Here are a few examples of prayers and blessings, from my satchel of sufficiencies.

When I was about ten years old, my family moved from my hometown of Omaha, Nebraska, to Tempe, Arizona. It wasn't long after that when my parents divorced. My "dad" soon found a new wife with a daughter of her own, then moved to North Carolina with his new family. My mom, brothers, and I moved in and out of apartment buildings over the next several years.

Arizona was hot, high school sucked; my brothers went their ways. Joe and Tony both married young and had babies early. My mom moved to Phoenix to be closer to her work. I was twenty- two years old. I had a lousy job, lived in a tiny apartment, and I had no chance at getting into college or ever paying the tuition. I just wanted to get the hell out of that miserable place.

On May 10, 1987, I loaded up my BMW 2002 with my golf clubs, some clothes, and my stereo, along with 1,800 bucks, all the money I had in the world at that time. I was committed to moving to California and never, ever looking back. I felt like Mr. Springsteen in "Born to Run." "It's a death trap, it's a suicide rap. We gotta get out while we're young!"

I remember loading one of my speakers into the car and accidently knocking the rearview mirror off the windshield. I tried to put it back into place, but I had broken the mount that held it to the windshield. I looked at that rearview mirror in my hand and said, "This thing is for looking backward. I'm not looking back, I'm moving forward." I threw the rearview mirror out the window and started out for California.

I knew no one in California. I had no place to live. I had no job, but I had 1,800 bucks, my good looks, my smile, the sound of my voice, and balls of an elephant. One other special advantage I had—my friend Eric. Eric got in the car with me and together we drove off into the Arizona sun toward the promised land of California. Eric suggested we go to his brother Mark's house in Leucadia. Maybe he would let me stay there for a couple of weeks until I could find a job and a place to live. Mark has always been a generous man, he was kind enough to let me stay for the rest of the month while I found a job and a room to rent in Pacific Beach.

Within thirty-five days of moving to California, I rented a room in Pacific Beach. I found a job, with LensCrafters. My BMW broke down under the La Jolla Village drive-off ramp. I left my car there and began to hitchhike when a lady in a white Ferrari picked me up and drove me all the way home. LensCrafters moved me from San Diego to Redondo Beach, then to Costa Mesa, where I became the youngest manager in the Western United States. Shortly after that I was offered a job to open a new store in Laguna where I met my future bride Shanna. Shanna and I have been married since 1991. Coincidence? Luck? Prayers and blessings.

In 1996, a few years later, I had started my real estate finance and investment firm. My son Julian had been born a couple of years prior. I had purchased my first home, business was growing, and I had a brand-new canary yellow Corvette.

One Saturday afternoon, I was driving my Corvette with my young son Julian to the San Diego Wild Animal Park. On the return home, I was also going to pick up an escrow check for $50,000 with my name on it. I was thirty-two years old at the time, doing well, new Corvette, beautiful son, and a fifty-thousand-dollar check in my pocket.

I called Shanna to let her know we were on our way home, hung up the phone, and proceeded to turn right to head home. BOOM! A fire truck ran over the hood of my Corvette. The fire truck skidded about a hundred feet before it came to a stop. Julian let out a yell that would curl your hair, a sound I had never heard before and never want to hear again. There was yellow fiberglass all over the street.

I got out of the car, ran to the other side to get my son. My heart was pounding, I was scared. Nothing happened to either of us. We were safe, completely unharmed after a 7,000-pound firetruck ran over the hood of my 2,300-pound fiberglass Corvette. I remember standing on the side of the road with Julian praying and thanking God that we were alive and uninjured. How does that happen? I remember thinking *pay attention!*

I thought I had the world by the tail and, in an instant, it could have been a deadly different outcome. My grandma always used to say, "We need more lerts around here, so be alert!"

The next day, we were in church and the sermon was on "the sound of your heavenly Father's voice." The pastor spoke on what he called a cage-rattling experience and how sometimes God will use a cage-rattling experience to get you to focus on Him. A fire truck running over the hood of my Corvette certainly rattled my cage. Were we just lucky? Was this some weird coincidence? More evidence of prayer and blessings?

A few months later, I met a man named Gary in the hallway of our office building. We introduced ourselves, shared some small talk about our respective businesses, and went on our way. A few days later, Gary stopped by my office and asked what I was reading. At the time I was studying Stephen Covey's book *First Things First*. I shared with Gary how I was working to grow a balanced life, intentionally growing myself mentally, physically, relationally, and spiritually. Gary suggested I read the Gospel of Luke, Chapter 2, verse 52, where it says Jesus grew in wisdom (mental), stature (physical), in favor with man (relational), and in favor with God (spiritual). Huh! How did he know that?

A week or so later, I was standing in Gary's office when I asked him about a diploma he had hanging on his wall. The diploma was a master's degree in divinity from Fuller Theological Seminary in Pasadena, California.

I asked Gary, "What does a master's degree in divinity mean?"

Gary looked at me, he looked at the diploma, looked again at me, and said, "Let's just say it is worth some level of respect."

I knew that I was in the presence of a man much wiser than me, so I asked him to teach me something. Gary asked what I wanted to learn. I replied, "Whatever it is that you think I should know."

Gary stated that he is a better teacher over a long period rather than a short period, then he told me to read the first chapter of the Book of Proverbs. I have been meeting with Gary every Monday morning since 1996. He has mentored me as we study the Word of God. How do you suppose that happened? Coincidence? Luck? Prayers and blessings.

I could write an entire book on how prayer has worked in my life and how God has blessed me as a result through experiences, relationships, and actual physical protection. I will share one more example.

On June 5, 2017, my son Julian was diagnosed with cancer. Over the next year, Julian would endure two major surgeries and 100 hours of chemotherapy. On November 9, 2017, only five months and four days later, I was diagnosed with cancer. Over the next year, I also endured two major surgeries and seven weeks of chemotherapy and radiation treatment every day, five days each week.

No one would willingly invite cancer into their life. The process is excruciatingly painful. We spent a tremendous amount of time in prayer and continue to do so. We have been blessed with many, many other people praying for Julian, me, and our whole family. Both Julian and I were fortunate enough to have been placed in the hands of the finest specialists in the world to treat us. We were both able to get our respective insurance companies to approve the specialists who were not in our "group." Our business was more profitable during this period than at any other time in the past.

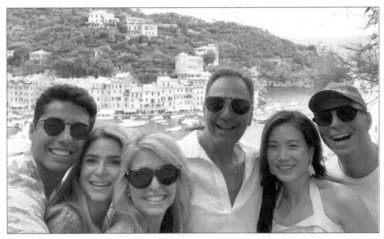

*Summer 2019, cancer free in Portofino with
the whole family, as promised. Sonny & Alexandra,
Shanna & me, Woo Jin & Julian.*

Today we are both cancer free. We exercise every day and are able to travel the world. Both of us have the opportunity to share with others in a positive way about our experience with cancer. If we hadn't had cancer, we would not have the authority to even speak on the subject, but because of cancer, we do.

Cancer has provided me the opportunity to write this book and encourage other individuals and families afflicted by this miserable disease. Cancer has opened unbelievable opportunities to share our faith and hope in Christ Jesus. The Book of James (named after me) in the Bible says "Consider it pure joy, my brothers and sisters, whenever you face trials of many kinds, because you know that the testing of your faith produces perseverance. Let perseverance finish its work so that you may be mature and complete, not lacking anything" (James 1:2–4, NIV).

People would never volunteer for this, but it does develop perseverance, it forces one to lean on God and it develops depth of character in an individual. It also comes with a deep level of responsibility. It is the individual's "ability to respond" and willingness to grow that develops into maturity not lacking anything. What a blessing!

## Lessons and Reflections

The education one receives at the University of Cancer is like no other education received anywhere in the world. Cancer will teach things nothing else can. I will share some of the lessons I learned during my time at the U of C.

The first lesson I learned is that I had cancer and didn't even know it. The only way I found out was because my son Julian had cancer. In some ways, his cancer might have saved my life. Had I not gone to urgent care with a cold while Julian was in his last week of chemotherapy, I might not have found out until the cancer had grown significantly.

I have always been a relatively healthy guy. In fact, I felt perfectly fine, even when I had cancer and didn't know it. Every year I would see my general physician for an annual check-up and share with him all the things I was doing to keep my body fit and as healthy as I could keep it. Dr. Vincent would tell me that I am the worst kind of patient he has, because I was doing everything right. He would tell me that there really is no rhyme or reason as to why some people live longer than others.

A mutual friend of ours used to drink a fifth of Jack Daniel's whiskey every day, smoke two packs of cigarette every day, scream and holler at everyone about everything, and lived to be in his nineties. Nothing could kill this guy! He finally passed away in his sleep with a smile on his face. Here I was doing what I thought was the best way to be healthy and live a quality life, and I got cancer at fifty-three years old. Julian got cancer at twenty-three years old!

Another clear lesson is that cancer doesn't care if you're skinny or fat, if you're rich or poor, if you're young or old, or what race or religion you are. Cancer does not discriminate; everyone is at risk and nobody really knows why. There is a whole legal industry attempting to blame anyone with deep pockets that their products or services cause cancer. Just ask Johnson & Johnson biotech company or ask Monsanto about its Roundup weed killer. These companies have been sued for hundreds of millions of dollars, and there is no clearly definable evidence that their products caused cancer. But there are big bucks in the business of who's to blame for everyone's problems.

The University of Cancer will provide a wonderful education about the insurance industry and how it works, or doesn't work, in your best interest. I have never been a fan of insurance companies because I generally believed that insurance companies are in business to collect premiums and not pay claims. In my battle and Julian's battle with our insurance companies, just trying to get to the best doctors to treat us convinced me that not only do they not want to pay claims, they are not interested in making sure you get the best care. They are interested in providing the minimal adequate and cost-effective care. Imagine how much worse it would be if the government oversaw the whole healthcare industry.

However, just as in every industry, there are good insurance policies, adequate policies, and poor insurance policies. Fortunately, we were able to get the best policies from the best insurance companies, and it made all the difference in the world—a life-and-death difference when dealing with cancer. The best insurance costs money and it's worth every dime. When a life is at risk, the cost of a quality insurance policy is insignificant to the value of that life. Get the best insurance from the most reputable company you can find and get one that is compatible with a Health Savings Account (HSA)! HSA plans are 100 percent deductible, just like an individual retirement account (IRA). Withdrawals to pay qualified medical expenses, including dental and vision, are never taxed. Interest earnings accumulate tax free and if used to pay for qualified medical expenses are tax free. (*Check with your insurance agent to see if you qualify.*)

It is sad that most people either can't afford the best insurance or don't know what type of coverage their adequate policy provides. It is no wonder that during every election cycle, health insurance is one of the primary policies that politicians argue over. Also, no surprise that insurance companies, healthcare providers, and pharmaceutical companies have the most powerful lobbyist and lobbying groups in Washington, DC.

Through my experience with cancer, I learned that there is a significant difference in the competence of physicians and nurses. Just because a person has an MD after their name does not mean they are a competent doctor, by any stretch of the imagination. And, insurance companies aren't going to any great effort trying to make sure you have the best care. You, as the patient, along with the help of your family, must do everything you can to make certain that the physicians who you are going to trust your life with are competent. This is a huge responsibility for a sick person, especially if you're sick with a deadly disease like cancer.

We were fortunate to have relationships with some influential people, and those influential people knew other influential people, and through those relationships, we are able to identify the best doctors and specialists to treat us. I traveled 170 miles each day, five days a week, for two months, to see the best doctors. I must have passed by dozens of hospitals and medical centers filled with thousands of the "wrong" doctors or less-than-the-best specialists.

One of my employees, Amber, lost her father to cancer in 2018. He had one form of cancer diagnostic, then a surgery that turned out to be completely unnecessary, then he was scorched so badly from radiation treatment that he had to be hospitalized again. Mike and his family endured five or six years of excruciating pain, procedures, and treatments. Ultimately, he ended up passing away at fifty-four years old. I am convinced that if he had received better care and a better specialist, he would be with us today.

Find the best doctors and specialists in the world and go to them, wherever they are and pay whatever the cost. Do not be afraid to get a second, third, or fourth opinion. As you do, the correct roadmap will begin to reveal itself, and you will know where to go and whom to work with. Option "B" is not an option; your life depends on it.

Another lesson I learned is that the human body is extremely resilient. I have had a robot in my mouth, surgically removing my infected tonsil, and a chunk of my tongue was chopped off with a surgical razor. I had my neck sliced open from behind my ear all the way under my neck and up to my chin. If you didn't know what I went through, you might have thought that the Mexican drug lord El Chapo Guzmán got me.

I had two cancerous tumors removed from my tonsil and thirty-one lymph nodes removed from my neck. I was sewn back together and sent home a few days later, only to return and endure seven weeks of chemotherapy and radiation treatments. Then I was hospitalized again because I was dying of dehydration. I was a mess, I looked like E.T., the Extra-Terrestrial and yet somehow, I survived. It is unbelievable what the human body can endure and recover from. I am not the same as I once was physically, but I am working on it.

The education I received at the University of Cancer is the type of education that people can't get from Harvard University or even Saddleback College; those places can and do teach theory. You can study theory all you want, but, in reality, all learning is in the "doing." As an example, read a book on how to play golf, or how to fly a plane, then go play golf or fly a plane, and you will quickly understand the minimal value of "theory."

The U of C teaches us through experiential application, "doing."

- We learn to deal with fear by dealing with fear.
- We learn resourcefulness by being resourceful and taking initiative.

- We learn resilience by being resilient.

- We learn responsibility by taking responsibility for our ability to respond to life-altering events.

- We learn to love in a way we never knew before, to love deeper with greater appreciation and forgiveness.

- We learn reliance by coming to the sobering conclusion that we cannot save ourselves and that we must rely on others.

This reliance includes doctors and healthcare workers to treat our ailments, family and friends to support us, employees to manage our businesses in our absence, and God to save us. He is the only savior and sooner or later each of us will turn to Him to rely on Him.

The Bible teaches us that "Every knee will bow before me; every tongue will acknowledge God" (Romans 14:11, NIV). You can either make that confession out of love and reverence, or you can make it out of fear and anger, but you will make that confession. It is entirely up to you. Life is precious and short; none of us get out of here alive.

## Graduation

As it is with all graduations, a new season begins. We are experiencing the completion of a difficult season and transitioning to a higher level. Graduation means you survived the hell called the University of Cancer, and you didn't do it alone. Your family and friends are all graduating along with you, as they too have shared in the journey.

It is a time to celebrate with all the doctors, nurses, and healthcare professionals who have helped you through this crazy season, while they remain to help the next graduating class. If you survive the season of cancer, you know that things will never be the way they once were, and you would be wise to embrace the lessons you have learned through the experience.

You can see the world in a whole new and beautiful way, with your eyes open to things you might have never recognized before. You will love like you never loved before, and you will forgive like you have never forgiven. Somehow, cancer will have made you a better you. You will have a different influence on those you love and especially other cancer patients.

I remember when Julian had cancer, and I would visit him during his chemotherapy treatments. I would try to encourage him and the other patients as they endured a process that was ravaging their bodies so that they could somehow heal. Most of these people would look at me like I had no idea what I was talking about, and they were right. There was no way I could possibly comprehend what they were going through.

However, when I was going through my chemotherapy treatments, it was different. I used to walk through the clinic with my six-foot, five-inch companion of dripping chemo-therapy bags and encourage other patients. Now, all of a

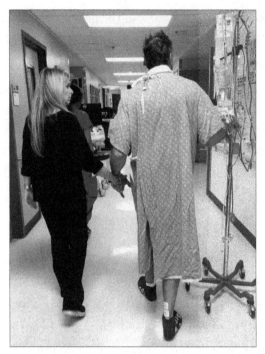

*Shanna and me walking the hallway
encouraging other cancer patients.*

sudden, I had something in common with them and I could comprehend what they were going through. I was one of them. I had a different authority, and they were much more receptive to my encouragement. Some were grateful and thankful, and some were belligerent and angry, which was understandable. Regardless, we all choose how we will respond in any given situation, including our response to cancer.

If you are fortunate enough to kill your own cancer by losing your life, you still graduate and begin a new season. In this too you will not be alone. All the doctors, nurses, healthcare workers, friends, and family will participate in this journey. It can be a painful and lonely experience for them. But love conquers all and soon a celebration of life takes place.

Dealing with death is a personal matter and your response can depend on your religion or lack of religion and your beliefs in life after death. Regardless of what you believe, death is an inescapable event, none of us will get out of here alive. Death will come, no matter what anyone might think. Accept it as a necessity; everyone will experience it.

The entire world is made up of only two elements, energy and matter; neither can be destroyed. Life is energy and like all forms of energy can be passed through various processes of transition or change. If death is not mere change, then nothing comes after death except a long eternal, peaceful sleep. Sounds good to me; everyone loves a deep and peaceful sleep.

Life is what we make it, always has been, always will be. Life's mysteries remain and deepen, its answers remain unresolved. So, we walk on through the darkness because that is where the next sunrise will be.

As songwriter John Mellencamp sings, "Oh yeah, life goes on, long after the thrill of living is gone."

Blessings,

James R. Perry

# ACKNOWLEDGMENTS

Acknowledgments can be lengthy; everything in life is built on meaningful relationships.

Clearly, I want to acknowledge my bride Shanna Lou, my son Julian, my daughter Alexandra, and their spouses.

I want to acknowledge the skilled and talented physicians who navigated me through this season in my life—Dr. Sinha, Dr. Bing, and Dr. Adam—and all the medical professionals at the medical center.

My staff at Alliance Portfolio for holding down the fort and keeping the business running in my absence.

All the prayers from those who prayed—you know who you are.

The collection of meaningful relationships I have developed. My family and closest friends, mentors, and employees.

To the publishing professionals—Ghislain who developed my cover art and book layout, Joni as editor and fellow Kansas City Chiefs fan. My publisher, printer, and marketing team, who assisted in making this idea come to fruition.

So many others who have played a part in my thought process, describing the experience in a way that will paint a meaningful picture to the reader.

If I am judged by the people I surround myself with, then clearly I AM A CHAMPION.

# ABOUT THE AUTHOR

JAMES PERRY IS PRESIDENT AND CEO of The Alliance Portfolio and managing member of Alliance Fund Management, LLC. Perry has specialized in placing private investor and pension fund capital into well-secured trust deed investments since 1989. He formed his first mortgage banking company in 1993, then cofounded The Alliance Portfolio in 1996. In 2007, Perry assumed complete ownership of The Alliance Portfolio and subsequently founded Alliance Portfolio Private Equity Finance in 2008. Perry has originated, funded, closed, and serviced over $700 million in private money trust deed investments. With over thirty years of experience, Perry has successfully navigated his and his clients' way through several real estate cycles, including the major market shifts in the early 1990s and 2007–2009.

Perry is an active member of the California Mortgage Association, where he is a frequent speaker, teaching classes on

"Raising Investment Capital," "Customers for Life—Effective Marketing Strategies," and "Marketing and Business Development." Perry is a sponsor of the Orange County Bar Association, Apartment Association of Orange County, Financial Planning Association of Orange County, and South Orange County Board of Realtors.

Perry is the author of *The University of Cancer: No One Applies; The Curriculum Can Kill You; The Education Priceless* along with *The Financial Planning Uses of Private Equity Real Estate Investments.* He has taught continuing education classes for the Financial Planning Association of Orange County.

Perry resides in San Clemente, California, with his bride of thirty years. He is committed to personal growth and actively works with a business coach, yoga and recovery coach, boxing coach, guitar coach, and spiritual mentor. He enjoys traveling to Italy and other beautiful spots in the world, playing golf, and studying business, leadership, and spiritual literatures.

### Connect with Me
E-mail: jperry@allianceportfolio.com

# PROCEEDS FROM THE UNIVERSITY OF CANCER

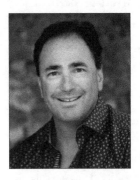

Years ago, a wise man shared with me a story about making a difference. He told me about a big storm and abnormally warm currents that swept along the Florida coastline. Thousands and thousands of starfish washed up on the shore and were dying on the sand. When the storm had calmed and the sun came out the following day, a boy was walking along the shore, picking up starfish and throwing them back into the ocean, giving the starfish a chance at life again. A man walking along the beach noticed the boy and asked, "Why are you throwing those starfish back into the ocean? There are too many; it won't make any difference." The boy looked at the man, reached to pick up a starfish and threw it back into the ocean. The boy said, "Made a difference to that one." (Adapted from "The Star Thrower" by Loren Eiseley, in *The Unexpected Universe,* 1969.)

While I was enduring my chemotherapy and radiation treatments, I met many other people who were experiencing the same treatments that I was going through. Many of them were driving a lot farther than I was. Many of them could not afford to stay the night in a hotel. One woman I met, Maria, was driving daily from Moreno Valley, some 200 miles one way in her 1991 Toyota Camry. She could barely afford gas to get her there and back every day.

The proceeds of this book will be used to help others going through cancer treatments. When I can give money to people like Maria, that will make a huge difference. If I were to give the proceeds of this book to a cancer organization, the proceeds would be diluted over so many people in need that the money couldn't possibly help anyone specifically.

So, the proceeds of this book will be used to make a difference in individual cancer patients' lives. I will seek the guidance of the doctors and the staff who helped me survive to recommend people who could most use the help to "make a difference in that one's life."

Blessings,

James Perry

CPSIA information can be obtained
at www.ICGtesting.com
Printed in the USA
LVHW080212050820
662290LV00013B/201/J